5 Steps to *Control* **High Blood Sugar**

Learn about

5 Steps to Control High Blood Sugar

Dr. ANJALI ARORA

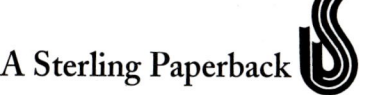

A Sterling Paperback

STERLING PAPERBACKS
An imprint of
Sterling Publishers (P) Ltd.
A-59, Okhla Industrial Area, Phase-II,
New Delhi-110020.
Tel: 26387070, 26386209; Fax: 91-11-26383788
E-mail: sterlingpublishers@airtelbroadband.in
ghai@nde.vsnl.net.in
www.sterlingpublishers.com

5 Steps to
Control High Blood Sugar
© 2007, *Dr. Anjali Arora*
ISBN 978-81-207-3243-8

All rights are reserved.
No part of this publication may be reproduced, stored in a retrieval system or transmitted, in any form or by any means, mechanical, photocopying, recording or otherwise, without prior written permission of the authors.

The author and publisher specifically disclaim any liability, loss or risk, whatsoever, personal or otherwise, which is incurred as a consequence, directly or indirectly of the use and application of any of the contents of this book.

The author wishes to thank all academicians, scientists and writers who have been a source of inspiration.

Printed and Published by Sterling Publishers Pvt. Ltd.,
New Delhi-110020.

Contents

1. Test Yourself for Diabetes — 8
2. Understand Diabetes Mellitus — 10
3. Measure Your Risk — 23
4. Diabetes and Lifestyle — 37
5. Diet, Exercise and Medication — 44

Myths and Fact File — 63

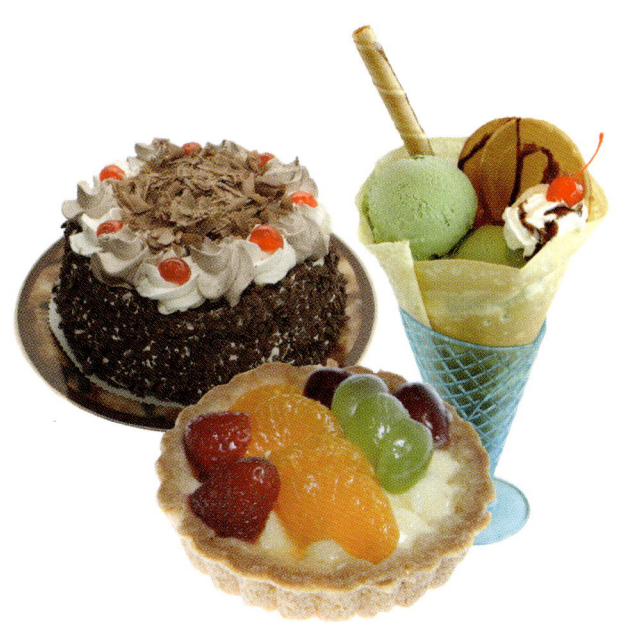

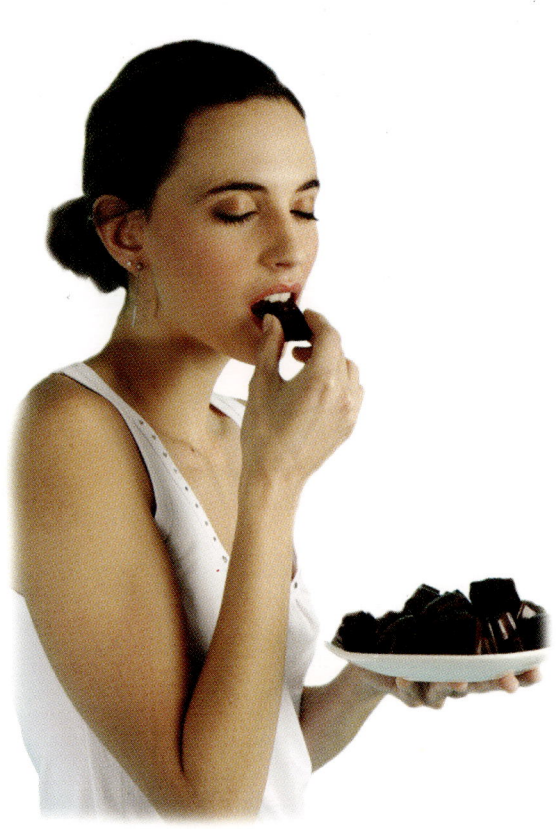

Diabetes or high blood sugar is a disease that occurs if there is a disorder in certain body functions that utilise carbohydrates, fats and proteins in the food to produce energy. Lack of a hormone called insulin or inadequate production of insulin by the pancreas results in this disease. Insulin regulates the amount of sugar in the blood. An imbalance in the amount of insulin produced can lead to the onset of diabetes mellitus.

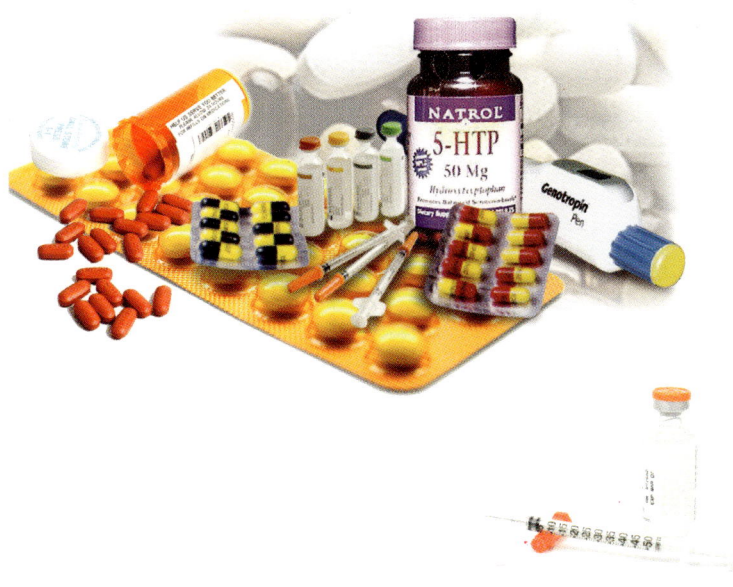

1   Test Yourself for Diabetes

Hunger and Thirst

Yes	No	
☐	☐	You are often very thirsty.
☐	☐	You feel hungry all the time.

Health Problems

Yes	No	
☐	☐	You have an itchy skin or skin problems.
☐	☐	You often develop boils.
☐	☐	Your injuries take a long time to heal.
☐	☐	You often get leg pain and cramps.

Urinary Problems

Yes	No	
☐	☐	You have to pass urine often in the day.
☐	☐	You get up at night to pass urine.
☐	☐	You frequently develop urinary infections.

Yes	No	**General Symptoms**
☐	☐	There is numbness or a tingling sensation in your feet or hands.
☐	☐	You have lost weight recently without making an effort.
☐	☐	You feel tired and weak.
☐	☐	You are very nauseous.

Yes	No	**Other Risk Factors**
☐	☐	You have a family history of diabetes.
☐	☐	You are overweight.

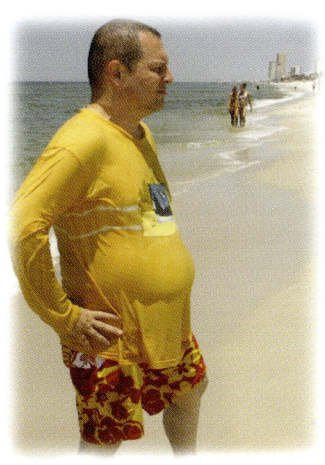

The more times you answer "yes" to the above statements, the greater you are at the risk of developing diabetes mellitus.

2 Understand Diabetes Mellitus

What is Diabetes?

Diabetes mellitus means 'honey sweet'. Diabetes occurs due to the inability of the body to convert food into energy. It is a condition where we have high blood sugar (glucose) levels in our body. It is a chronic disease, which can be managed well through proper guidance.

The Insulin Factor

Normally our body converts the food we eat into sugar or glucose, which is used for the production of energy. This is done by the pancreas, an organ lying near the stomach. The pancreas makes a hormone called insulin, which attaches itself to the receptors on the cell wall, thereby allowing glucose

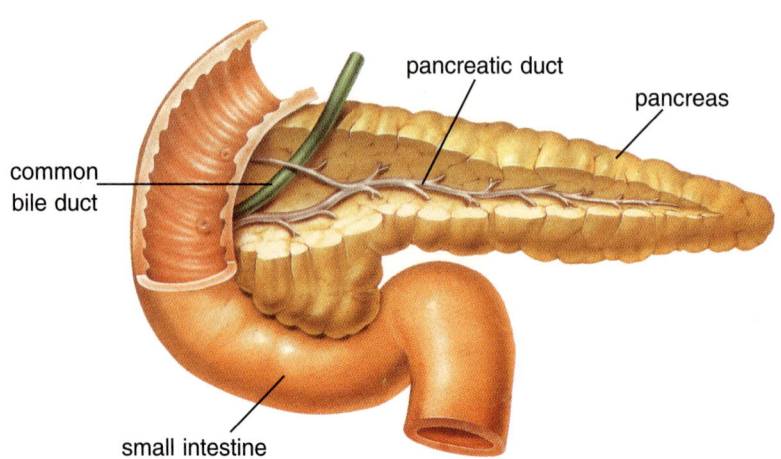

to enter the cells. It acts as the key, unlocking the receptors for glucose to enter the cells. The cells then metabolise the glucose to give energy to the body.

Insulin Resistance

The pancreas makes enough insulin, but due to certain factors, the insulin is not effective in transferring glucose from the blood into the cells of the body. Such a disorder is referred to as insulin resistance.

Factors involved can be:

- The number of receptors on each cell becomes lower than normal.
- Insulin is not able to attach itself to the receptor.
- Insulin produced may be defective.

With the passage of time, the capacity of the pancreas to produce insulin declines.

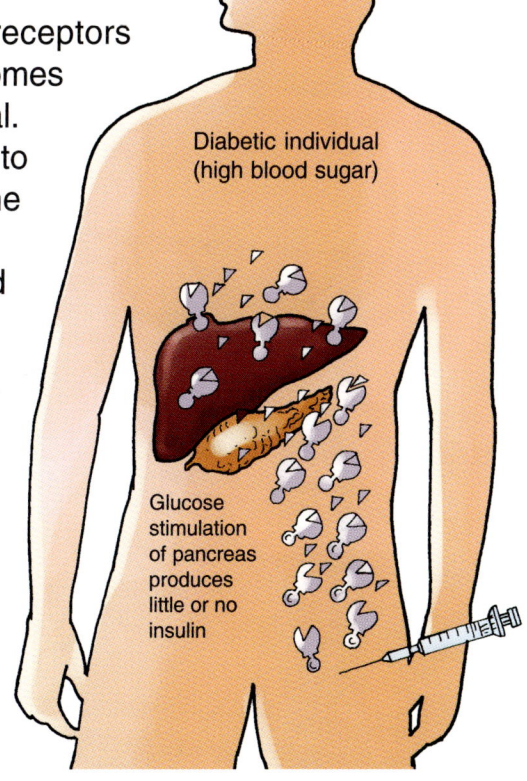

Diabetic individual (high blood sugar)

Glucose stimulation of pancreas produces little or no insulin

Types of Diabetes

Type I Diabetes

Type I diabetes is a severe form of disease. It is an auto-immune disease, which mostly develops in childhood or in adults under 30 years of age.

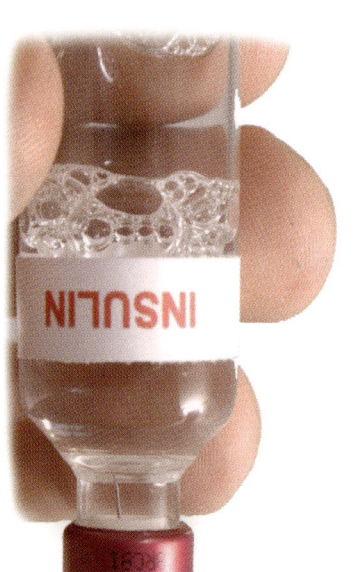

(Auto-immune is when the body's immune system starts destroying itself) 'Juvenile diabetes' develops in childhood and must be treated with insulin. It accounts for 5-10% of diabetics in the world.

Inside the pancreas are cell clusters known as the

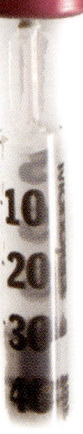

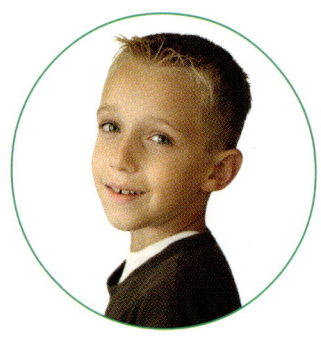

islets of langerhans. There are several type of islet cells including alpha cells and beta cells. Insulin is produced by beta cells. On increase of sugar in the blood, these cells manufacture insulin and then release it into the blood stream. The role of these cells is to monitor levels of blood sugar. In people withType I diabetes, beta cells are attacked by the immune system and are destroyed slowly. What exactly causes the immune system to get affected is still based on a number of theories. The unfortunate part is that, though this slow destruction takes place over a number of years (5-7), the symptoms of diabetes mellitus do not surface until about 80% of these beta cells are destroyed. Eventually, insulin production comes to a halt as no beta cells remain.

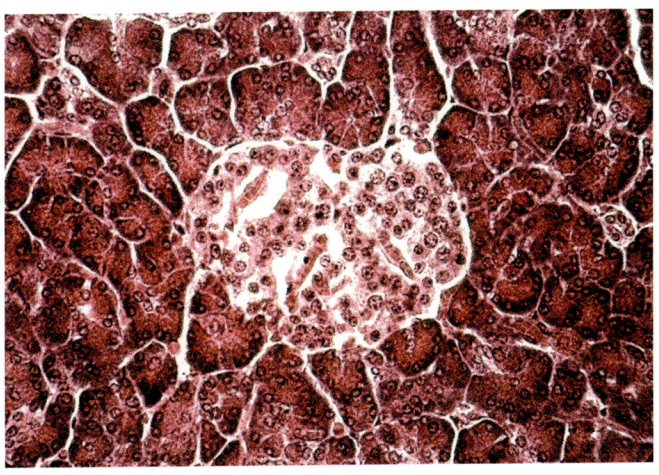

Islets of langerhans

Theories on the Development of Type I Diabetes

- **Genetic Predisposition :** Genetic predisposition determines entirely whether a person will develop immune reactivity against insulin producing β-cells in the pancreas. However environmental factors and infections can have a major impact on whether Type-I diabetes will manifest itself clinically. This occurs after 80-90% of the β-cells have been destroyed. The remnants of β-cells are transported to the pancreatic draining lymph node (PDLN), where the ensuing auto immune is thought to be coordinated. Debris from the β-cells is picked up by Antigen-Presenting Cells (APC) and displayed to immune cells called lymphocytes (L) prompting them either to kill β-cells or to signal further immune reponses.

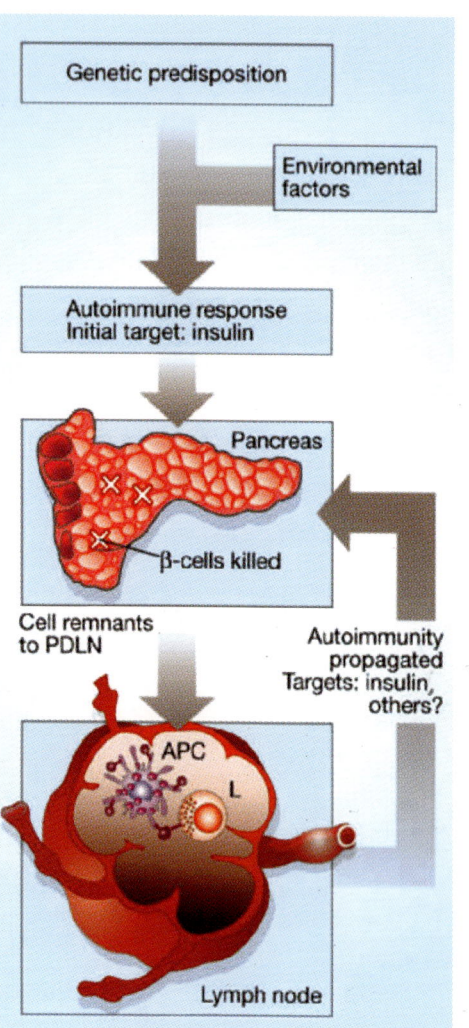

- In Type I diabetes, the body loses the ability to make insulin, as the immune system destroys the insulin-producing cells.
- When insulin is not available, the glucose remains in the bloodstream and cannot be used as energy.
- A person having Type I diabetes has to take insulin injections to stay alive.

- Virus Infection
- Cold Weather

The Thrifty Gene Theory

This theory was proposed by J. A. Neel in 1962. It suggested the reason as to why Indians suffered from a disproportionate high rate of Type II diabetes. According to him, Indians lived a hunter gatherer existence for centuries. For their survival, they developed a gene which allowed them to survive the cycles of feast and famine. Their metabolism was adequate in itself in both these conditions, it utilised the calories efficiently.

With an unstable food supply, their survival was better as they could somehow store surplus energy (in the form of fat) during the time of feast. This fat was probably stored as abdominal fat and utilised during famines.

Exposing this gene to abundance of food continuously in the present environment in all likelihood is proving to be detrimental.

Diabetic Ketoacidosis

Ketoacidosis develops mainly in people with Type I diabetes. This disease is the result of persistently high levels of blood sugar (hyperglycaemia).

Blood sugar builds up in the body as your cells cannot absorb glucose for energy. The glucose not available to the body, starts burning body fat as fuel, thus producing waste products called ketones. This accumulation of ketones in the blood is known as ketosis.

When these ketone bodies are excreted in the urine the process is called ketonuria. The increase of ketones in the body over a course of some days leads to fluid being depleted from the body in the form of urine. This results in dehydration leading to the pH of the blood becoming acidic. The process of ketoacidosis sets in. Unrecognised and untreated ketoacidosis can lead to coma and death.

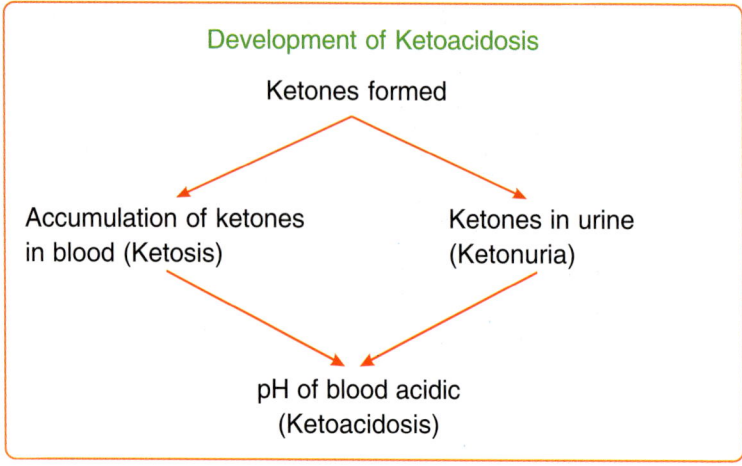

Symptoms of Ketoacidosis

- Frequent urination
- Great thirst
- Nausea and vomiting
- Blurred vision
- Drowsiness and disorientation

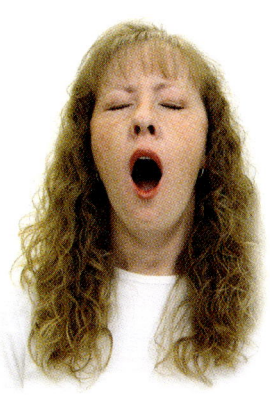

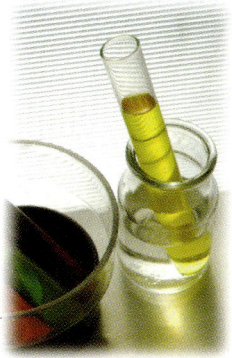

To Detect Ketoacidosis

If your blood sugar levels are over 200 mg/dl for two consecutive tests, test your urine for ketones. Ketones also known as acetones can be detected in the urine by the acetone test.

Ketoacidosis and Coma

If a person goes into coma due to ketoacidosis, it is a serious situation. Mild ketoacidosis does not lead to coma. It is only when the ketone bodies are present above a certain level that coma occurs. Any of the symptoms mentioned above and the presence of ketones in the urine are an indication of administering insulin when blood sugar is high.

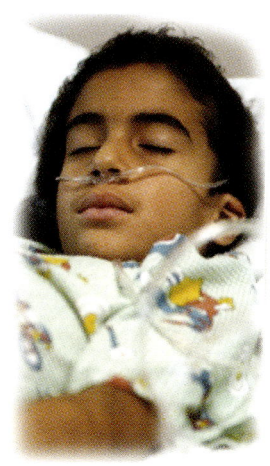

Type II

Type II diabetes is often called non-insulin dependent diabetes mellitus.

This type of diabetes develops in adulthood. It develops due to less production of insulin or ineffective use of insulin. This form of diabetes is present in 90-95% of diabetics in the world. Women during their pregnancy can develop a form of Type II diabetes called gestational diabetes. 40% of women with gestational diabetes during pregnancy develop Type II diabetes within four years.

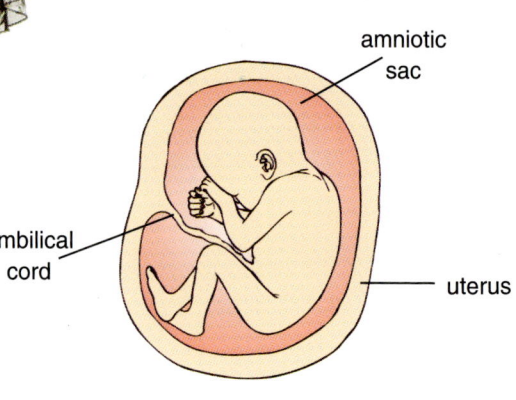

Human Foetus

Impaired Glucose Tolerance

Impaired glucose tolerance is a term when blood sugar levels are higher than normal, but not high enough to be diagnosed as diabetes mellitus. This impairment is indicated by a fasting glucose reading ranging between 100 and 130 mg/dl. The symptoms relating to diabetes mellitus are normally absent. If a person reduces his risk factors, his impaired glucose tolerance may improve.

Blood sugar level therefore may become normal or stabilise. Some people with impaired glucose tolerance may go on to develop diabetes.

How Does Diabetes Mellitus Develop?

Due to malfunctioning in the production and utilisation of insulin, the amount of glucose produced remains in the bloodstream, causing high blood sugar or hyperglycaemia. In turn, the cells do not have enough blood sugar to provide the energy required.

Some Common Terms in Diabetes

Hyperglycaemia is high blood glucose or sugar.

Symptoms

- Tiredness
- Thirst
- Nausea
- Blurred vision
- Frequent urination
- Dry itchy skin
- Genital itching

Hypoglycaemia is low blood glucose or sugar.

Symptoms

- Shakiness
- Irritability
- Confused state
- Pounding heart
- Sweating
- Light-headedness
- Hunger pangs

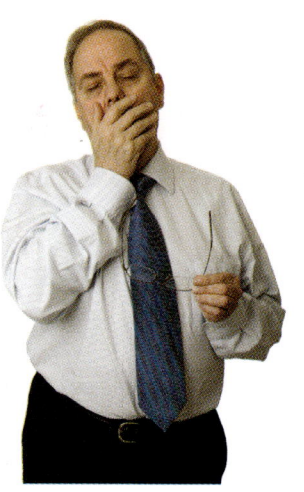
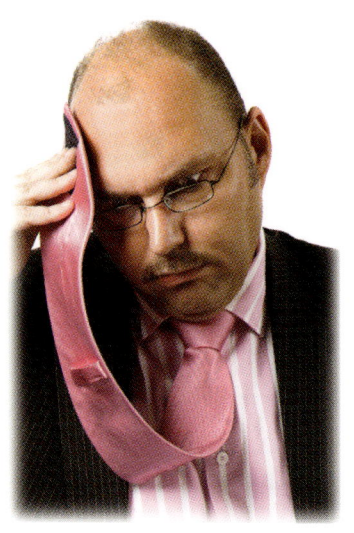

Factors Causing High Blood Sugar (Hyperglycaemia)

- Eating food containing simple sugars which are rapidly absorbed by the body, e.g. sweets, ice creams and pastries.
- Drinking sweetened beverages such as carbonated drinks and juices.

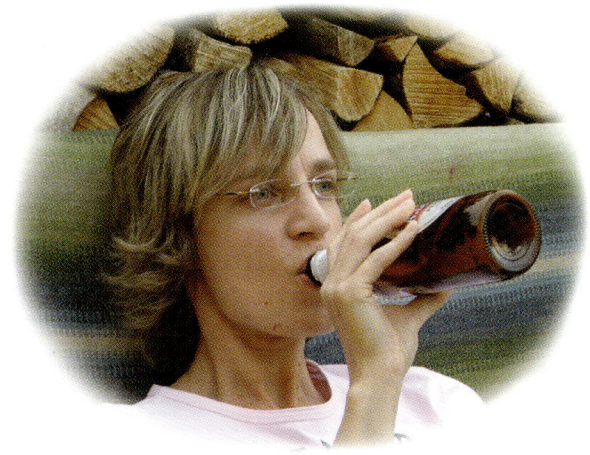

- Sedentary lifestyle – not burning the consumed sugar, carbohydrates and other products.
- Not enough administration of insulin or other medication.
- Physical stress (e.g. infections, flu).
- Psychological stress.

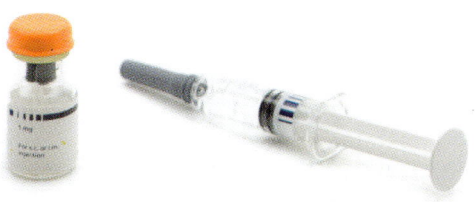

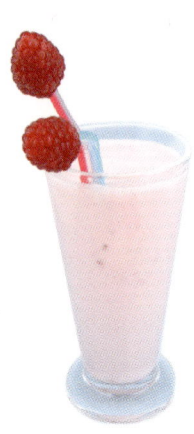
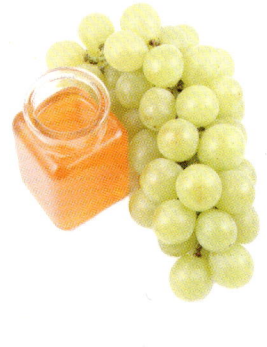
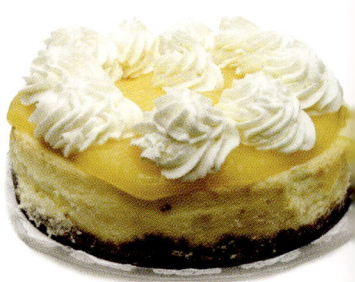

Factors Causing Low Blood Sugar (Hypoglycaemia)

- Skipping or delaying a meal.
- Taking too much of insulin or diabetic medication.
- Not taking enough carbohydrates in a meal.
- Sudden increase in exercise.

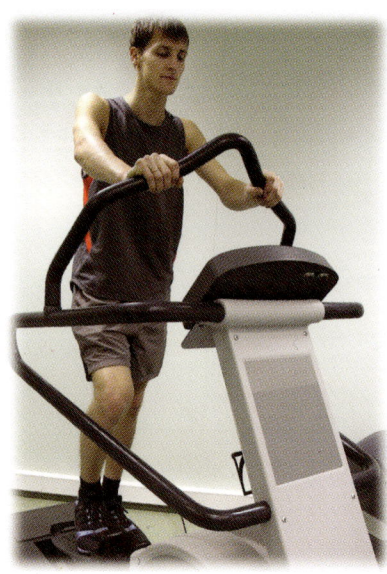

3 Measure Your Risk

A few simple tests can help determine whether you have diabetes.

The Venous Sample Test

This is done in the laboratory. It can be of four types: fasting (F), postprandial (PP), glycosylated haemoglobin and oral glucose tolerance test (GTT). Except for postprandial, all the other tests should be done 12 hours after an overnight fast, without even a cup of tea.

Fasting: The normal fasting blood sugar level is less than 100 mg/dl. If your reading is higher than this, a diagnosis indicative of developing diabetes is made.

Postprandial: The postprandial is conducted 2 hours after a heavy meal or after taking 75 gm of glucose. A reading of over 130 mg/dl along with other positive tests, is indicative of diabetes.

Glycosylated Haemoglobin Test: HbA1c is a measurement to assess the level of your blood sugar over the past 120 days. An HbA1c reading of over 6.1% is suggestive of diabetes.

Oral Glucose Tolerance Test: After fasting overnight, you are given water with 75 gm sugar (in a water-sugar solution). Your blood glucose levels are tested over a 24-hour period.

In a diabetic person, blood glucose levels rise higher than normal and do not fall as quickly. A normal blood glucose reading, two hours after drinking the solution, should be less than 130 mg/dl. All readings between zero to two hours should be less than 200 mg/dl.

In addition to these, a random blood sugar reading can be taken any time. A reading of above 140mg/dl can be indicative of diabetes.

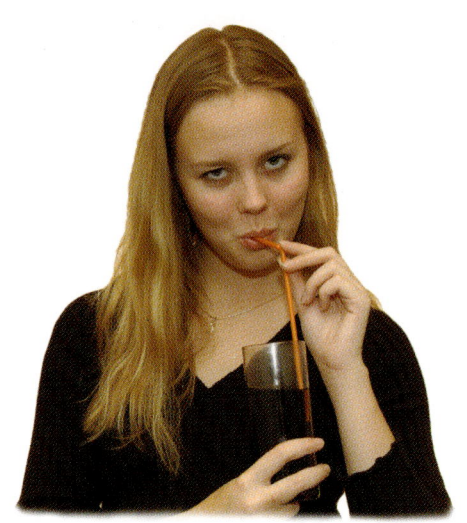

The Single Stick Blood Glucose Test

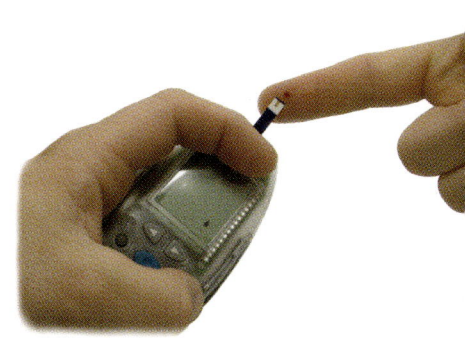

The finger is pricked with a needle. The blood sample is placed on a strip. The strip is then placed in the slot of the glucometer machine, which assesses your blood sugar level. This method is to be used only to monitor your blood sugar levels at home. It is not completely reliable, so a venous sample should also be assessed in the laboratory as guided by your doctor.

Urine Test

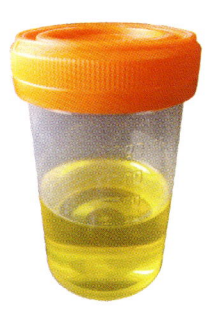

You may also be advised by your doctor to get a routine sample of urine tested for albumin, sugar and microalbuminurea.

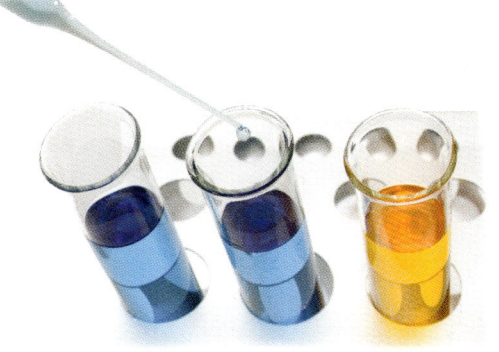

Screening for Diabetes

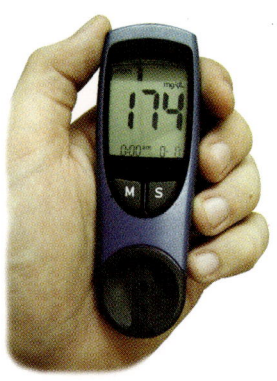

This should be done at 30 years of age. If a history of heart attack, stroke or diabetes prevails in the family, then a blood sugar test should be done along with a lipid profile at 20 years of age to determine the person's baseline level. The tests can be repeated every 3 years if normal. If abnormal or borderline, tests should be repeated annually or as your doctor advises.

Risk Factors for Developing Type II Diabetes

- A person having a parent or sibling with Type II diabetes.
- If a person is overweight or has high blood pressure, he or she is at a greater risk of developing diabetes.
- A person having high levels of cholesterol and triglycerides is at a greater risk of developing diabetes. With diabetes and abnormal fat levels, a

person increases the risk of heart disease up to four times in comparison with the general population.

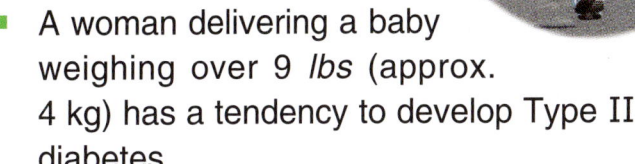

- A person having a sedentary lifestyle has greater chances of developing diabetes. This risk can be reduced by exercising regularly.
- A woman delivering a baby weighing over 9 *lbs* (approx. 4 kg) has a tendency to develop Type II diabetes.
- If a person's blood sugar levels are regularly above normal then he or she is becoming a prediabetic and will probably become a diabetic within 10 years.
- Continuous stress is today known to be a predisposing factor for developing diabetes mellitus.
- A family history of Type II diabetes (particularly in a first-degree relative) in presence of other risk factors can precipitate the development of diabetes.
- Ethnic groups (Asian or Afro-Caribbean) are more prone to develop diabetes.

- Previous history of gestational diabetes or previous diagnosis of impaired glucose tolerance, can both lead to the development of diabetes mellitus.

Diabetes Mellitus and Obesity

Overweight and obese people keep producing the hormone insulin, but it cannot act appropriately. An obese person having a high carbohydrate intake puts a strain on the body's glucose metabolism. Also, obesity reduces the insulin receptors on the surface of the cells. As the uptake of insulin is less by fewer receptors, the body's sensitivity to the insulin is reduced.

Cells (mainly fat or muscle) requiring glucose, cannot get it from the blood. There is a famine in the midst of plenty, resulting in diabetes.

In response to the high blood sugar present, the pancreas works more to produce more insulin. Eventually, this constant pumping of the pancreas exhausts the pancreatic beta cells. Insulin secretion from the pancreas starts becoming inadequate and overweight people become diabetic.

Diabetes Mellitus and LDL Oxidation

In diabetes mellitus, LDL is glycosylated by the process of glycosylation, i.e. attachment of sugar to LDL-C. This modified LDL-C makes it stick to the arteries, thus enhancing the process of atherosclerosis and heart disease .

Secondary Diabetes

It can occur due to a number of causes:

- Hormonal abnormalities
- Insulin receptor disorders
- Pancreatic disease
- Drug induced diabetes
- Corticosteroid administration
- Genetic syndrome

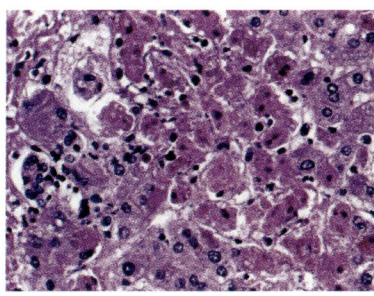

Diseased Pancreas

Studies show that if there is even 1% reduction in HbA1c (glycosylated haemoglobin) in diabetics then:

- The risk of microvascular complications (e.g. in kidney, eye) is reduced by 37%.
- The risk of fatal and non-fatal heart attack is also reduced by 14%.

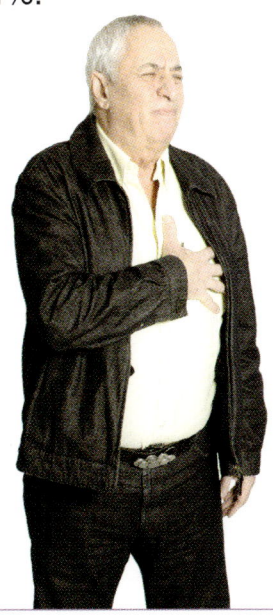

Diabetic Complications

High Blood Sugar

High blood sugar levels over a period of time can lead to major health problems.

- Blood vessels can get affected, leading to heart attack, stroke and circulatory problems.
- Frequent urinary infection is due to the presence of high sugar (not well controlled) which results in the damage of the kidneys.
- Kidney disease (nephropathy) may result, which often leads to end-stage renal disease and kidney failure.

The Kidney Malfunction

Just as the kidneys lose their ability to discharge wastes, they also lose their ability to retain protein and sugar. Sugar and protein are detected in urine tests often in large amounts. Blood tests detect high levels of urea, nitrogen and creatinine which indicate damaged kidneys.

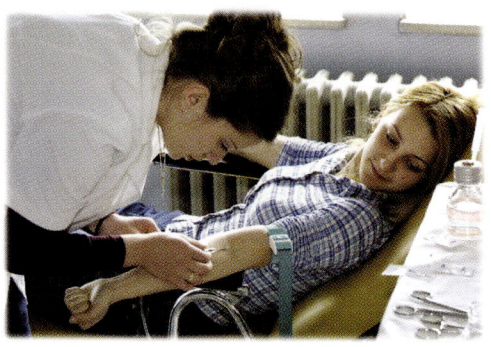

Effects of Kidney Malfunction

- If kidney damage (nephropathy) progresses, a person may have to undergo kidney dialysis. Kidney transplantation might also be an option. High uncontrolled blood sugar can also lead to neuropathy.

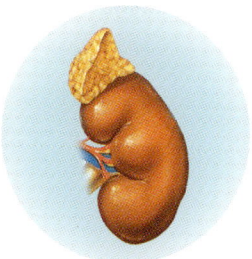
Human Kidney

- Nerve problems (neuropathy) may occur, causing a 'pins and needles' sensation in the hands and legs.

- Diabetes damaging the nerves can also lead to reduced pain or loss of sensation in the feet. Skin sores or ulcers on the feet can be a result of bad footware.

Ulcer in the Foot

- Injuries or infections do not heal well. Often an injury on the foot does not heal and can lead to gangrene.

Diabetic Retinopathy

It can result due to some disease or damage to the small blood vessels of the retina. Eye problems get complicated and can result in retinopathy, premature cataract and glaucoma. Retina is the area of the eye on which the image (picture of what we see) is formed by our lens system. People with long standing diabetes often develop this disease.

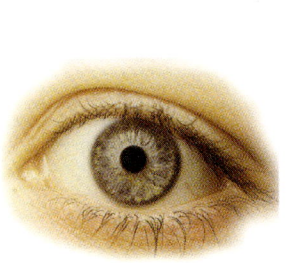
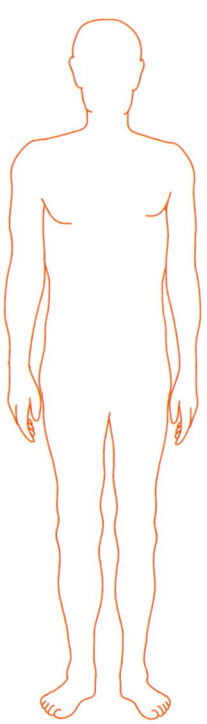

Diabetic Retinopathy Causes Damage to Small Blood Vessels of the Retina

Skin Disease

- **Diabetic Dermopathy:** It is the commonest kind of skin disease seen in diabetics. Skin develops brown scars over the shin of legs. This is due to abnormal changes in the small blood vessels of the skin. If diabetes is not kept under control, the process of ageing gets faster.

Blood Glucose, Lipids and Blood Pressure Control

This is a part of diabetic care. It is important to reach target levels mentioned below. Failure to do so would lead to a deteriorated lifestyle.

Blood Glucose Control and Microvascular Risks Involved

	Low risk	Arterial risk	Microvascular risk
HbA1c %Hb	<=6.5	>6.5	>7.5
Venous plasma glucose fasting mmol/l mg/dl	<=6.0 <110	>6.0 >=110	>=7.0 >125
Self-monitored blood glucose fasting mmol/l mg/dl	<=5.5 <100	>7.5 >=100	>=6.0 >110
Postprandial mmol/l mg/dl	<=7.5 <135	>=7.5 >=135	>9.0 >160

Blood Lipid Control and Risk Levels with Diabetes

	Low risk	Medium risk	High Risk levels
Serum total cholesterol mmol/l mg/dl	<4.8 <185	4.8-6.0 185-230	>6.0 >230
Serum LDL cholesterol mmol/l mg/dl	<2.5 <100	2.5-3.3 100-130	>3.3 >130
Serum HDL cholesterol mmol/l mg/dl	>1.2 >46	1.0-1.2 39-46	<1.0 <39
Serum triglycerides mmol/l mg/dl	<1.7 <150	1.7-2.2 150-200	>2.2 >200

Assessment of blood glucose, lipids and blood pressure should be done as follows:

- Glycosylated haemoglobin assayed between every two to six months.
- Blood lipid profile to be assayed between every two to six months (If border line is high).
- Blood pressure measurement on each consultation.

(lower risk being: <140<85 mmHg)

For the "tight" blood pressure group (a mean BP of 144/82 mmHg), there was a reduction of risk of diabetes-related deaths (32 per cent), stroke (44 per cent) and in all the other diabetes-related end points. Also, the risk of myocardial infarction was reduced.

Some More Statistics

- There are over 32 million diabetics in India.
- Every eighth Indian is a diabetic.
- 95% of these diabetics suffer from diabetes mellitus II.

According to the World Health Organisation, India is predicted to be the diabetic capital of the world by 2030, harbouring 79 million diabetics.

Food, Hormones and Body Balance

Some Facts

- Your body has a limited capacity to store carbohydrate and protein.
- Your muscles and liver together cannot store more than 1800 cals of carbohydrate. After this capacity is filled, food is converted into fat.
- A continuously sustained rhythmic form of exercise for about 45 minutes helps burn fat.
- Any food consumed affects your insulin and glucagon secretions.
- When you eat carbohydrate in your food, your blood sugar level rises, stimulating insulin secretion. This insulin gets the tryptophan–serotonin mechanism working in the brain. The feeling of pleasure or feeling good is a result of this serotonin production in the brain.
- A recent study states that diabetics consuming 50 gms of natural fibre in their daily diet, lower their glucose level by 10%. It was seen that a high fibre diet also helps decrease insulin levels in the blood. In patients of diabetes mellitus II, lipid levels also get lowered with the fibre. Consumption of soluble and insoluble fibre containing fruits, vegetables and grains is beneficial.
- Chromium, a trace mineral, plays an important role in insulin sensitivity. Its deficiency also promotes an imbalance in glucose metabolism.

For a good body-mind balance it is important to have an even secretion of insulin. Roller coaster secretion leads to excessive mood swings, hunger, stress, cholesterol and fat deposits.

Foods Helpful in Controlling Blood Sugar Levels

Source	Form	Action
Bitter Gourd (Karela)	Cooked vegetable or juice with seeds grounded.	Helps reduce blood sugar levels.
Fenugreek Seeds (Methi Dana)	Soak a teaspoon of *methi* seeds in water overnight. Swallow them in the morning with water.	Supportive in controlling diabetes.
Black *Jamun*	Fruit or *jamun* powder	Janboline in the *jamun* helps control blood sugar levels.
Spirulina	Leaves or dried powder	Helps stabilise the blood sugar levels.
Low fat curd	Butter milk (*chaach*)	Stimulates pancreas to produce insulin and helps control blood sugar.
Primose plant	Plant supplements	Helps balance blood sugar levels.
Chana Dal	Sprouted	Helps in utilising glucose in the body.

All these products are supportive in controlling diabetes mellitus. A balanced diet, exercise and prescribed medication should not be neglected.

4 Diabetes and Lifestyle

General Guidelines

- Avoid fatty, junk, fried and preserved foods.
- Try and lose weight if you are overweight.
- Have more high-fibre foods and complex carbohydrates.
- Choose healthy snacks.
- Take your prescribed medication regularly.
- Monitor your blood sugar regularly.

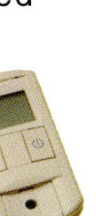

Glucometer

DIABETIC CHART		
Date	Time	Medicine

- Be active, but check with your doctor before doing strenuous exercise.

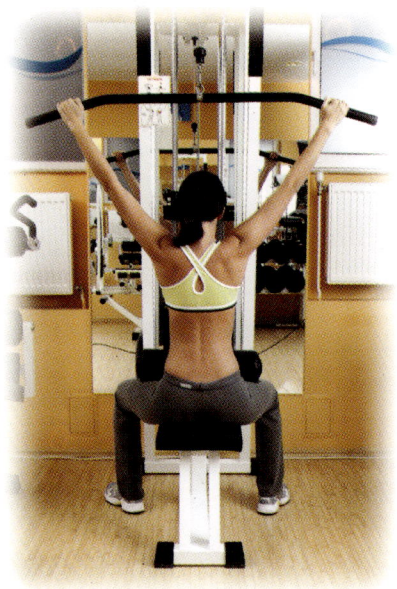

- If you follow a regulated lifestyle, you can indulge a little occasionally!
- Avoid alcohol. It has empty calories. If necessary, drink in strict moderation.

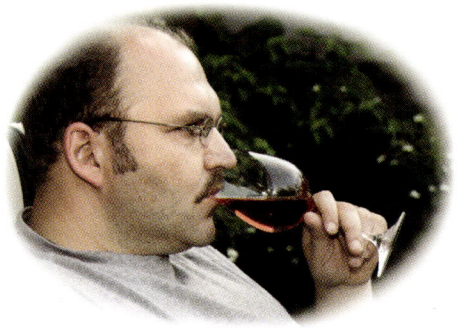

- Follow an organised routine.
- Eat the same amount of food daily.
- Eat at about the same time daily.
- Exercise at the same time daily.

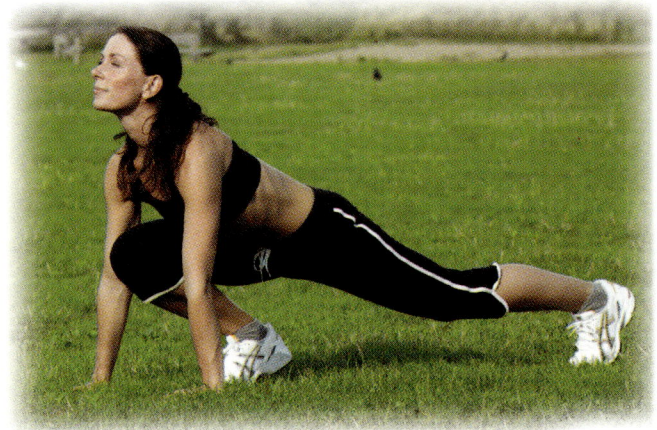

- Take your medication at the same time daily.
- Avoid stress. Destress yourself with massage, yoga or meditation.
- Don't miss a meal. If you travel frequently and have long eating gaps between meals, carry sweets or toffees to avoid hypoglycaemia.

Monitoring of Blood Glucose Level

Self-monitoring should be done by every diabetic who is concerned about managing their disease. It is especially recommended for anyone using insulin, whether having Type I or Type II diabetes.

Monitoring is important as...

- An identical dose of insulin will be absorbed differently from day-to-day.
- It also depends on factors such as exercise, stress, type of food taken and an individual's insulin sensitivity.
- Hormonal changes in a woman (e.g. puberty, the menstrual cycle and pregnancy) are also factors involved with insulin absorption.
- Self-monitoring of insulin dosage is also recommended when a different (new) type of insulin (company or dosage) is administered.

Blood glucose monitoring is also recommended to patients on a oral hypoglycaemic drug. This is recommended to avoid hypoglycaemia (low blood sugar), especially if the diet has been less or the patient has been vomiting and suffering from diarrhoea.

Diabetics and Illness

It is important to keep your blood sugar under control when you are ill.

- Drink lot of water.

- If you cannot eat your regular food, have sweetened lime juice, crackers or soup. You need calories to avoid hypoglycaemia.

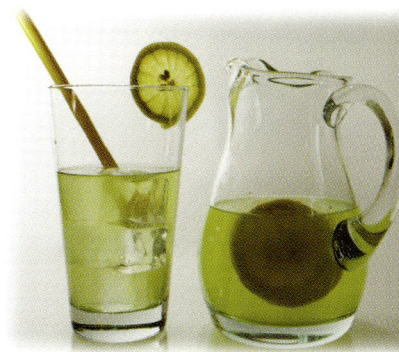

- Keep taking your diabetic medicines as advised.
- Monitor your blood sugar.
 It may still be high, even if you are not eating regular meals.
- Consult your doctor if you have vomited or are having diarrhoea.

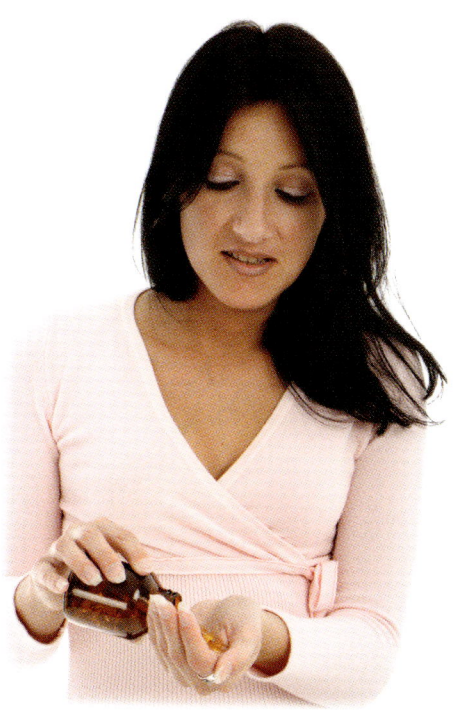

Injuries and Foot Care

- Do not walk barefoot to avoid foot injury.
- Minor injuries, cuts or infections should immediately be attended to.
- Foot care is of extreme importance. After having a bath in tepid water, pat your feet dry with a clean towel, especially between the toes.
- Check your feet regularly for any cuts or bruises or rough cracks in winter. Prevent infections by applying antiseptic cream immediately. Consult a doctor for any lingering infection.

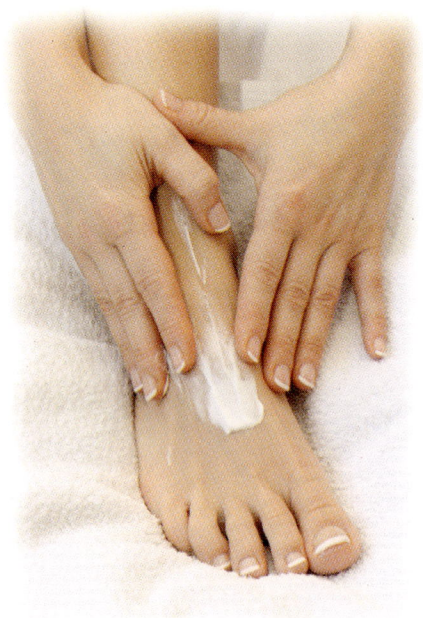

- Wear clean cotton or woollen socks which are comfortable and not skin irritants.
- Wear leather or sports shoes which are not tight fitted. Be careful of shoe bite.
- Do not use hot water bottles or heating pads near your feet.
- Avoid cutting your toe nails too close to the skin. File them straight slightly rounding the corners.

Dental Care

Uncontrolled diabetes increases your risk of gum disease, caries and development of more cavities. Regular dental care (brushing or flossing the teeth after every meal) is important in people with high blood sugar. Dental check ups should be done as advised by your dentist.

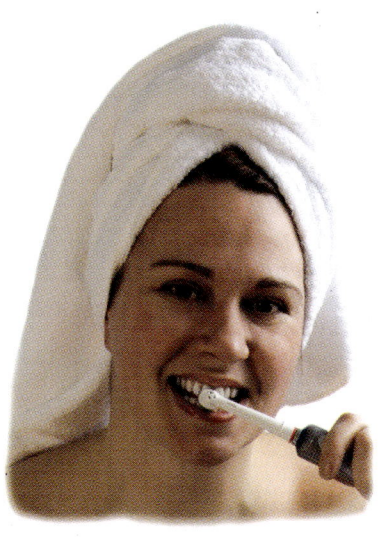

5 Diet, Exercise and Medication

People having diabetes mellitus II can control their disease with the help of the following.

- Diet
- Exercise
- Weight loss
- Medication

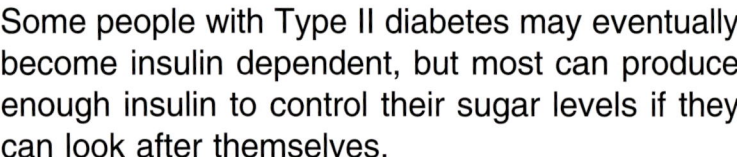

Some people with Type II diabetes may eventually become insulin dependent, but most can produce enough insulin to control their sugar levels if they can look after themselves.

Diet

The diabetic meal should consist of high fibre, low fat and protein. Fruits and vegetables are rich in minerals, vitamins and antioxidants and therefore should be consumed. Salads can also be freely taken by diabetics, but with limited use of oil.

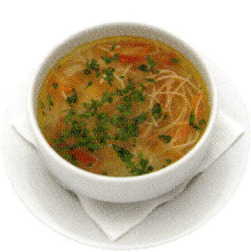

Total proteins: 15-20% of calories required.

Fats: less than 30% of calories required.

Carbohydrates: 55-60% of calories required.

Fibre: 25 gms per day for women, 40 gms per day for men (approximately).

Diet Schedule

Main Meals
- Breakfast ✓
- Lunch ✓
- Dinner ✓

Snacks
- Mid-morning ✓
- Evening Tea ✓

> A diabetic must have three main meals and two sugar-free snacks every day.

A complex high-fibre carbohydrate diet is recommended for diabetics. Also known as starches, complex carbohydrates are slowly absorbed, thereby keeping blood sugar levels fairly stable. Examples are wholewheat products, brown rice, beans, oats, vegetables and fruits.

- To increase your fibre intake, high fibre breakfast cereal (with no sugar) can be consumed.
- Eat more vegetables. Increase the amount of beans, peas, nuts and other pulses in your daily diet.

- Go for small amounts of food. If overweight, try cutting down the calories you consume in a day.

Some Useful Food Tips for Diabetics

Rice

The calorific value of rice is very close to cereals like wheat. Rice, unfortunately on consumption increases blood sugar levels rapidly. Therefore, rice should be consumed in small quantities. It is also important to consume rice in combination with oats, whole wheat bread, dals (lentils) and vegetables. The high fibre content present in these foods helps prevent a rapid increase in blood sugar levels. Unpolished or brown rice is a better dietary option than polished rice.

Sugar and Sweets

Sugar or sweet consumption is not directly related to the development of diabetes mellitus.

Inability of the body to produce insulin leads to diabetes when the body is unable to utilise sugar or carbohydrate. On consuming sugar, in a person prone to diabetes mellitus, there is a substantial increase in blood sugar levels leading to diabetes or aggravating the existing condition.

Actually, excessive consumption of sweets leads to weight gain. Weight gain in combination with sedentary habits, family history of diabetes mellitus and stress are the precipitating factors for developing diabetes.

Fruits and Fruit Juices

Diabetics can consume fruits but in limited quantity. *Jamun*, sweet lime, papaya, guava, strawberry, apples, and oranges can be taken by diabetics as they have fibre and minerals. Also, these fruits release blood sugar gradually in the body. Banana, mango, chiku, grapes (the sweet fruits) are to be eaten once in a while and that too in small quantities.

Fruit juices should not be taken by diabetics as instant sugar is released and there is also no benefit of fibre.

Healthy Cooking Techniques

Low-fat food can be tasty, healthy and enjoyed by your whole family when you use healthy cooking techniques such as boiling, baking, stewing and roasting.

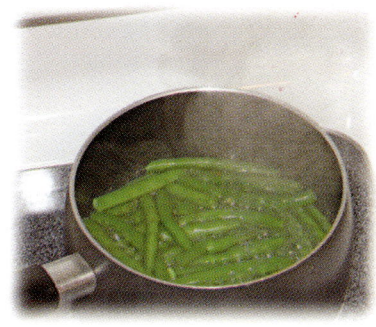
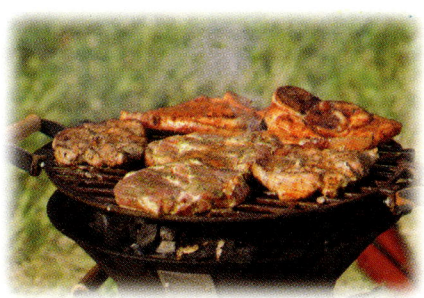

- Microwave, broil, grill, stir fry, boil, barbecue or steam food with minimal salt or fat.
- Cook on a low flame.
- Use non-stick cookware.

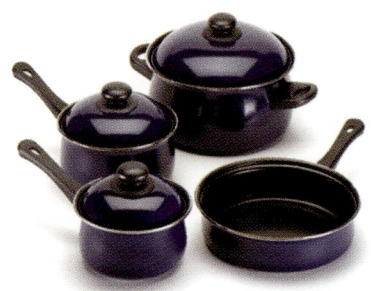

- Try and have low-fat recipes.
- Favour the use of monounsaturated fats (mustard, olive, rapeseed oils) and polyunsaturated fats (sunflower and safflower oils) in place of too much saturated fat (palm oil). Blend two or more oils for healthy cooking.

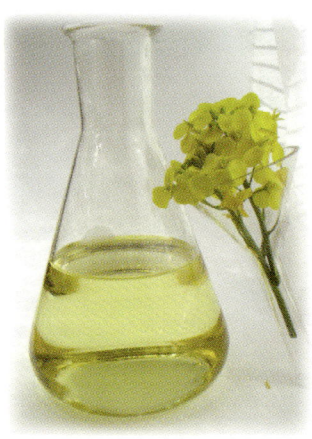
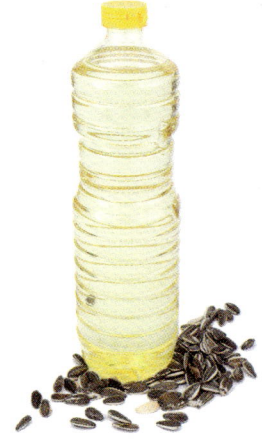

Healthy Ways to Consume Vegetables

- Use low-fat or fat-free salad dressings.
- Cook or steam vegetables using very little water. Overcooking will break down the fibres.
- Season food with chopped onion, garlic, tomato or lime juice.

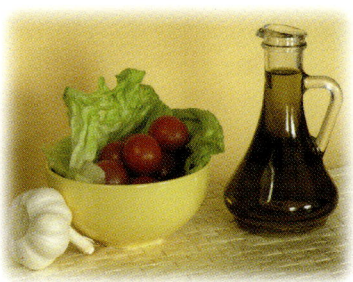
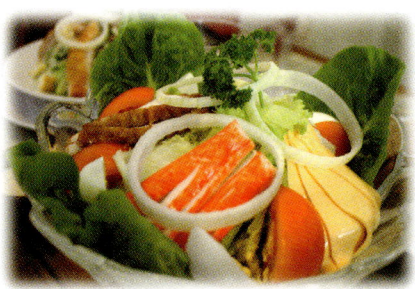

Healthy Ways to Consume Fruits

- Consume raw fruits. Do not peel fruits like apples and pears.
- Eat small portions and only consume the amount required in your diet.
- Eat fruits instead of drinking fruit juice (which gives you only sugar and no fibre).

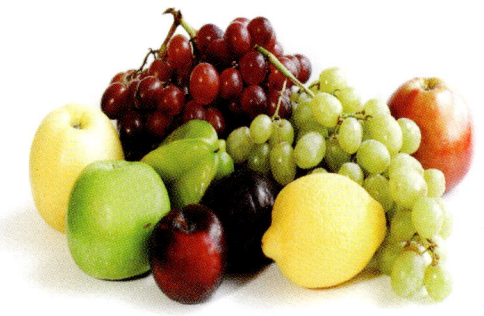

Healthy Ways to Consume Milk and Milk Products

- Drink skimmed or non-fat or low-fat milk.
- Consume low-fat or fat-free yoghurt (curd).
- Make cottage cheese out of fat-free or low-fat milk.

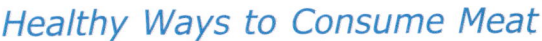

Healthy Ways to Consume Meat

- Eat more of fish.
- Cook chicken without the skin.
- Buy meat with less fat.
- Trim off extra fat as far as possible.
- Avoid fatty meats like bacon, mutton and sausages.
- Have egg white.

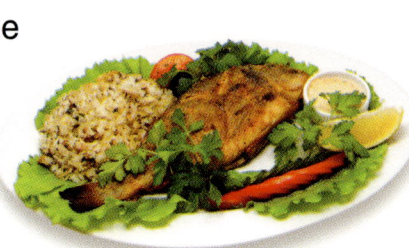

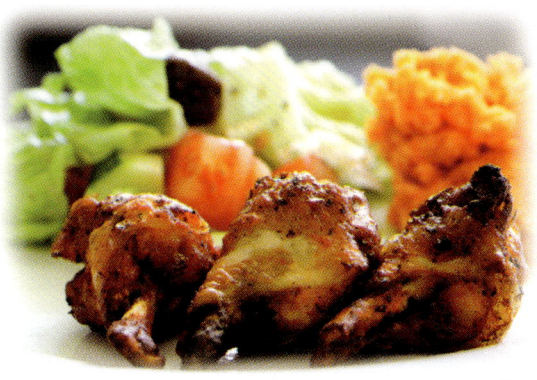

- Flavour your food with lemon juice, soya sauce, vinegar or herbs.
- Limit the use of condiments like mustard, ketchup and salad dressing (they are high in salt or sugar).

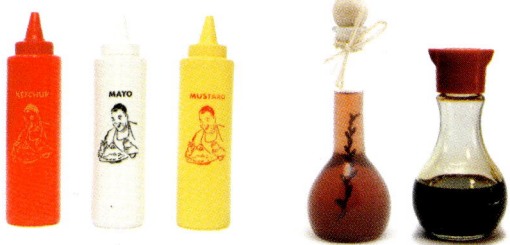

Artificial Sweeteners

Sugar substitutes are saccharin and aspartame. Saccharin is calorie free. Aspartame has negligible calories per serving. They can be used instead of sugar. All artificial sweeteners should be used to the minimum.

Exercise

- Test your blood sugar levels before exercising.
- If your blood sugar levels are not too high, have a small snack 15-20 minutes before exercising.
- Don't inject insulin into that part of your body which you will be exercising. It gets absorbed faster from there.
- While exercising, watch out for signs of hypoglycaemia.

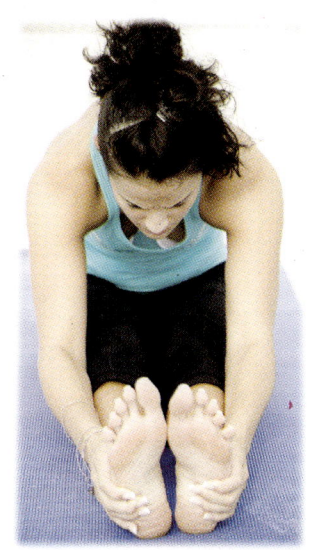

Benefits of Exercise for Diabetics

- **Less restrictive diet:** Exercise burns calories. You can eat reasonably well and still keep your blood sugar and weight at a healthy level.
- **Less insulin required:** Exercise helps in increasing the body's sensitivity to insulin and burns glucose more efficiently.

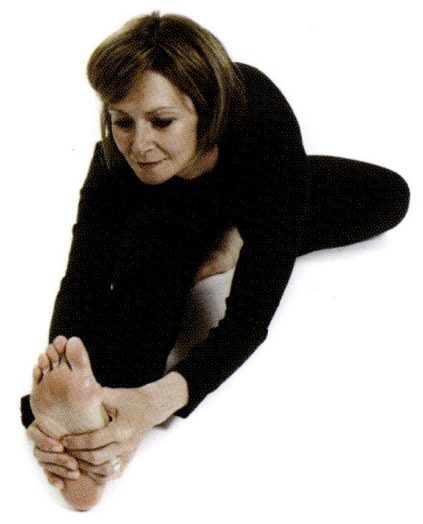

Calories burnt by an individual in ½ hr with the following weight

Exercise type	50 Kg	60 Kg	75 Kg
Walking	105	125	155
Jogging	225	245	275
Swimming	190	230	290
Cycling	150	180	240
Exercising (Moderately)	150	170	200

Diabetic Food Pyramid

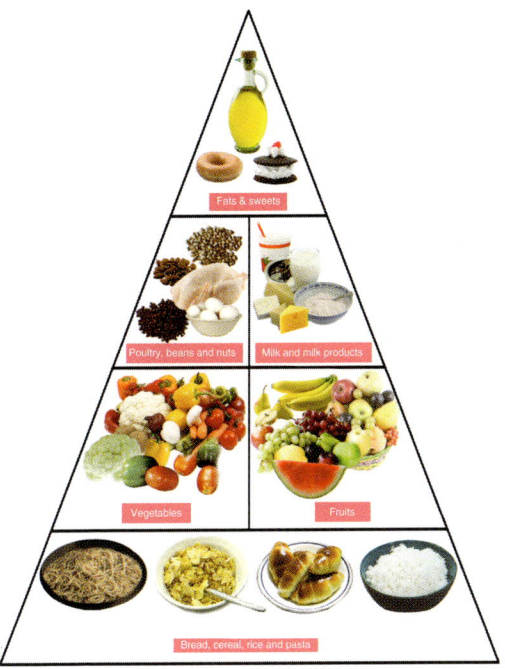

Medication

After getting your blood sugar reports, consult your doctor for the type of medication you require. Type I and Type II diabetics require different kinds of medication. Also, factors such as whether you are obese or thin, or have other medical problems besides diabetes will decide the dosage and the group of medicines to be taken.

Medication for Diabetes Mellitus

Oral antidiabetic agents are used for patients of non-insulin dependent diabetes mellitus (NIDDM II).

These patients should be administered this medication after they have been put on a restrictive carbohydrate diet. Administration of medication should be along with proper diet and exercise.

Biguanide (Metformin): It is the medication of choice today. Its action is to primarily increase the peripheral uptake of glucose. In large doses, it also helps to decrease the intestinal absorption of glucose.

Sulphonylureas (Gilbenclamide, Glimepiride and Glipizides): They produce hypoglycaemia by stimulating the release of insulin. They also help inhibit the release of glucose by the liver and increase the sensitivity of peripheral tissue to insulin.

Thiazolidinediones (Roziglitazone and Pioglitazone): They help enhance sensitivity to insulin in the liver, adipose tissue and skeletal muscle.

Post Prandial Glucose Regulators (Repaglinide and Nateglinide): They help stimulate the release of insulin from pancreatic beta cells.

Alpha Glucosidal Inhibitors (Acarbose): When taken with a meal Acarbose reduces the post prandial glucose peaks by retarding the glucose uptake by the intestine. Acarbose can be administered as a monotherapy or in combination with other hypoglycaemics.

Insulins: They are prepared as bovine, procine or human insulin. Insulin preparations are classified according to their duration of action. The more common ones are:
- Short acting insulins
- Intermediate and long acting insulins

Insulins are normally administered to patients of IDDM. The recent concept is to also put patients of NIDDM on insulin as to avoid complications of diabetes later.

All diabetic medications can have side effects. No diabetic medication whether for NIDDM or IDDM should be taken or administered without the doctor's prescription.

Site for Insulin Injection

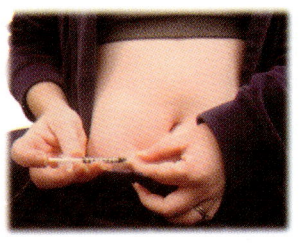

The most common site for an insulin injection is the abdomen. The back of upper arms, the upper buttocks or hips and the outer side of thighs are also used as insulin injection sites. These sites are good for injecting insulin because:
- They have a layer of fat just below the skin to absorb the insulin.
- Not too many nerves are present in that area making it more comfortable compared to other parts of the body.

Easily Available

- Reasonably priced, easy-to-use home glucometers are available.
- Insulin pens, which can be carried in the pocket, are easy to administer and cause minimum discomfort to the patient.
- Also available are insulin pumps, which can be inserted under the skin.

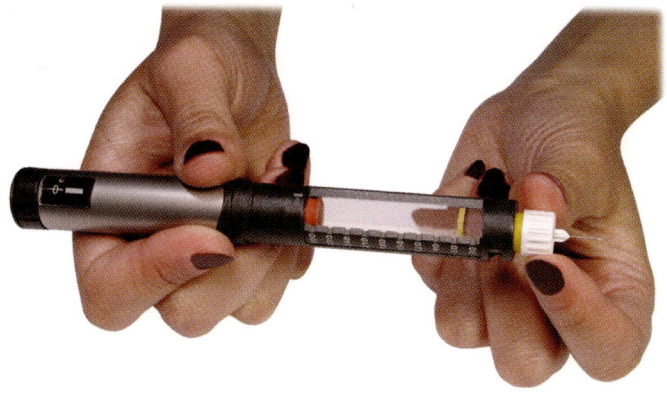

- Diabetic jam, flour, chocolates and ice creams are available at many outlets.

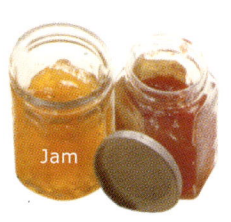
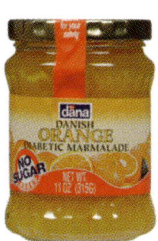
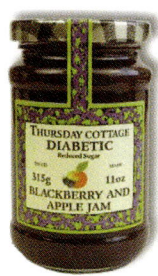

Advancements in the Treatment of Diabetes

Diabetes is one of the most common diseases affecting people worldwide. By 2010, India is expected to become the World's Diabetic Capital. In the United States, it has affected an estimated seventeen million people. Today we have come a long way since insulin's discovery in 1921.

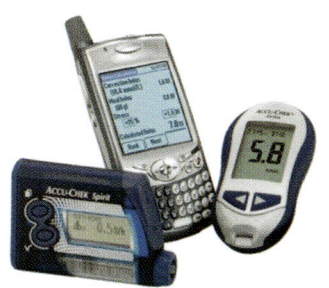

Smart Meters

They help to regulate food intake, exercise, medication, blood glucose readings and weight, all with push-button ease.

Alternate Site Testing

Finger tips are the easiest site for drawing a sample for blood glucose testing. The new tester (freestyle) offers the opportunity to draw a blood sample from an alternate test site.

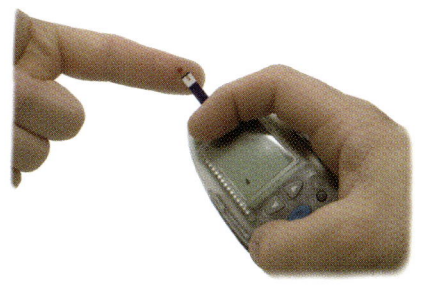

Home Testing

The glycated haemoglobin test is now available as a single use fingerstick test with results available within minutes.

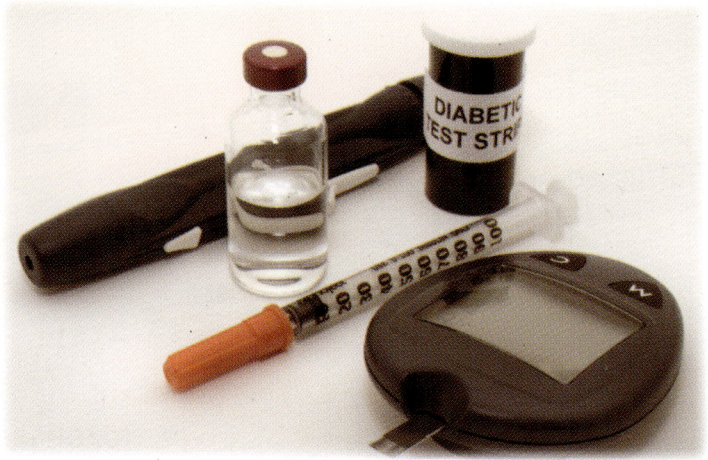

While a fingerstick provides a glucose level for a moment in time, the glycated haemoglobin level reflects the glucose level in the body for the most recent two to three month period.

Non-invasive Glucose Monitoring

It is a well-established fact that people with diabetes who closely monitor and regulate their glucose levels have fewer complications from the disease. A recently developed device "GlucoWatch G2 Biographer" will make glucose monitoring easier. The Biographer is a glucose-monitoring device that looks like a watch. It is completely non-invasive and uses a low electrical current to pull fluids through the skin. It then measures the glucose level in the fluid.

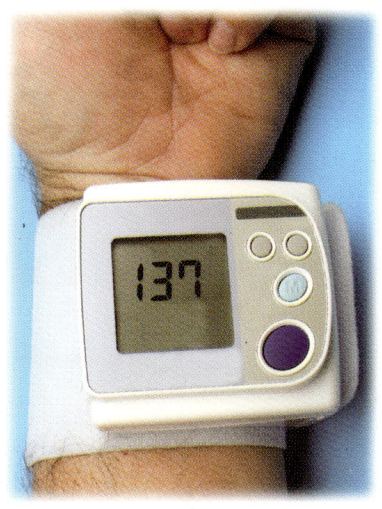

The watch can be worn for up to 13 hours and can test glucose levels as often as every ten minutes. This does not eliminate the need for standard fingersticks. The hope is that devices like these will eventually make them unnecessary.

The Biographer can also show people how their bodies react to specific situations like exercise, stress, meals, sleep, and medications (all of which can affect glucose levels). There is an alarm on the watch that can be set to go off if glucose level becomes too high or too low.

Insulin Pump

The most recent device, to be introduced, is a wireless insulin pump system. The system is called the Medtronic MiniMed Paradigm 512 Insulin Pump and Paradigm Link Blood Glucose Monitor. It comprises of a glucose monitor, external insulin pump, and dose calculator that work together to determine the amount of insulin needed.

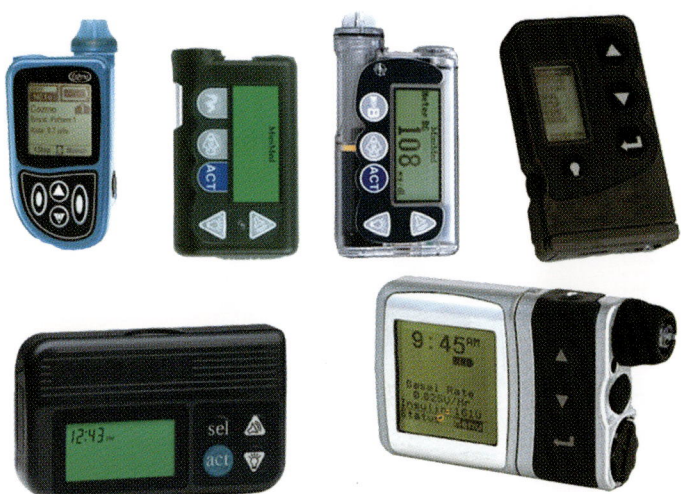

On the Horizon

There are many new treatments being studied to improve the lives of people who have diabetes. Insulin is being studied in new forms including longer acting doses. New modes of delivery are also being examined including

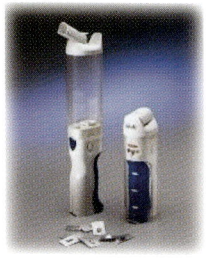
Diabetic Inhalers

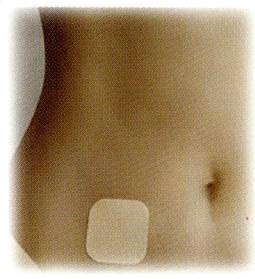
Diabetic Skin Patch Test

inhalers, *skin patch*, and *oral insulin*. Other medications under investigation hope to enhance the release of insulin from the pancreas in order to balance glucose levels (by regulating other related hormones), and treat complications of diabetes.

Pancreas Transplant

A pancreas transplant is a surgery to implant a healthy pancreas from a donor into a patient with diabetes. Pancreas transplants give the patient a chance to become independent of insulin injections.

Partial Pancreas Transplantation

When a patient with diabetes receives a kidney transplant from a living relative, it is usually beneficial to perform a partial pancreas transplant at the same time. Since the transplanted kidney will become damaged by diabetes over the time, transplanting a partial pancreas from the same donor will help control blood glucose levels and protect the new kidney from further damage.

Benefits and Risks of Pancreas Transplants

- Pancreas transplants are safest in people who do not have heart or blood vessel disease.
- The healthier you are, the better you can withstand the physical stress of surgery.
- Immunosuppressive drugs are important and hard on the body. People who have to undergo a pancreatic transplantation should avoid those who have infections, such as a cold or the flu. They should not be immunised without first checking with their doctor. These drugs can also damage the kidneys.

A successful pancreas transplant can benefit a Type I diabetic person in at least three ways:

- Some amount of diabetes-related damage to the body can be controlled.
- Insulin injections are no longer needed and the person can enjoy a regular diet.
- A person can enjoy greater activity and independence.

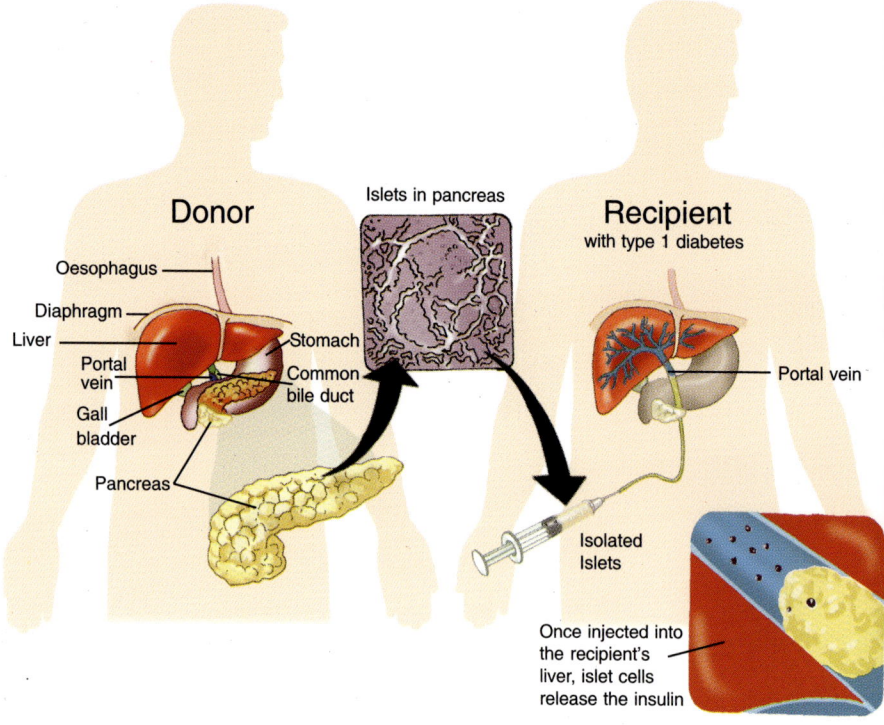

Pancreas Transplant

Myths and Fact File

Myth

I do not have a history of diabetes in my family. I will never develop it.

Fact

Genetically you are less prone to developing diabetes. However, because of sedentary lifestyle, wrong eating habits, excess weight and stress, one can develop diabetes mellitus.

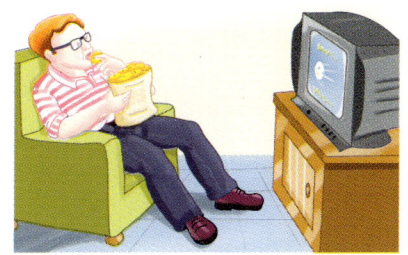

Myth

Alcohol does not affect diabetics adversely.

Fact

Consumption of alcohol can worsen the disease. It can also react with the given diabetic medication.

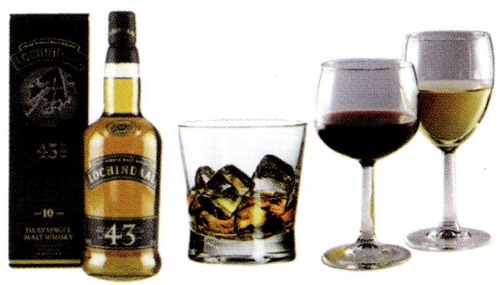

Myth

As a diabetic, I get tired easily, so I should rest.

Fact

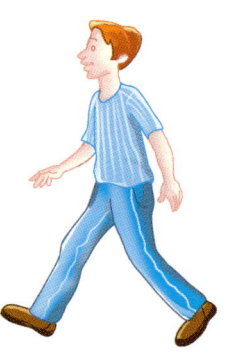

Diabetes should be kept under control. All diabetics must be active and have a regular exercise routine. However, exercise must not be strenuous.

Myth

Diabetics cannot eat any fat or carbohydrates.

Fact

Diabetics should have a minimal amount of fat and mostly keep to monounsaturated or polyunsaturated fats. Complex carbohydrates with less calories and more fibre can be taken.

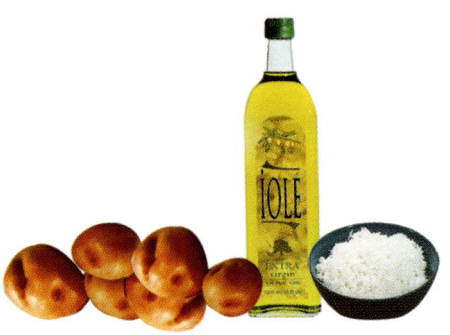